VALTER LONGO FOUNDATION

NUTRITION
BEGINS AS CHILDREN

Manual for Families and Teachers

WELCOME

to the manual for families and teachers of "Nutrition Begins as Children", a creative and educational coloring book.

This manual offers valuable support that integrates the coloring book with engaging activities that promote fun and interactive learning.

Let's explore together the infinite ways of using this educational tool!

* The author's proceeds, generated by the book 'Nutrition Begins as Children' by the Valter Longo Foundation, are intended to support research and non-profit projects promoted by the Foundation itself, which aim to promote nutrition education in schools and to provide nutritional assistance to people in particularly critical financial and health situations.

TABLE OF CONTENTS

1. THE VALTER LONGO FOUNDATION

The Valter Longo Foundation was founded in Italy in 2017 by Professor Valter Longo, Ph. D, Director of the Longevity Institute of the School of Gerontology at the University of Southern California (USC) in Los Angeles and Director of the Oncology and Longevity Program at the IFOM Institute of Molecular Oncology in Milan, Italy. Professor Longo was included by the American magazine "Time" in the list of the 50 most influential people of 2018 in the health sector and is known throughout the world for the creation of the "fasting-mimicking diet" and for his global best-seller "The Longevity Diet". In 2021 the American scientific journal "Science" defined him as a pioneer in the field of nutrition and cancer.

The Valter Longo Foundation is a non-profit organization that aims to promote, implement, and optimize healthy and sustainable longevity for oneself, for others, and for the environment. This path towards longevity and health begins in childhood and continues throughout the entire life cycle. The goal is to create a balanced lifestyle and be able to live as well as possible so as to prevent various types of serious diseases, including tumors, diabetes, obesity, cardiovascular, autoimmune diseases - such as Crohn's disease and multiple sclerosis - and neurodegenerative diseases such as Alzheimer's.

The mission of its founder and the Foundation is to offer everyone, without distinction, the opportunity for a long and healthy life. To achieve its institutional objectives, the Foundation dedicates its daily efforts from, both a preventive and therapeutic point of view to:

1. the promotion, financing, and direct and immediate provision of health and social assistance, as well as nutritional consultancy, based on proven scientific data, The goal is a) to treat, prevent, or support people suffering from various diseases and living in a particular emergency condition or psychological, physical, and economic distress; b) to offer guidance to all those who wish to pursue healthy longevity;

2. raising awareness and educating the public of all ages on issues related to nutrition and a correct and healthy lifestyle based on scientific data.

2. INTRODUCTION AND CONTENTS OF THE MANUAL

The coloring book **"Nutrition Begins as Children"**, created by the Valter Longo Foundation (www.fondazionevalterlongo.org) in collaboration with the artist Manuela Lupis, is a book in **English and Italian** designed for primary school children, with a particular focus on the age group between 6 and 8 years, yet **accessible to a broader audience** to learn the principles of:

1. **A healthy lifestyle**

2. **Balanced nutrition**

3. **Physical exercise**

4. **Essential values for a long-lived, healthy, and sustainable life for oneself and others, such as sharing and a sense of community.**

In addition, it can be used by any age group **for those who wish to learn Italian or English as a second language.**

This book provides an enjoyable educational experience for children, complemented by a **manual** that offers support for adults, families, and teachers. It guides them on an **engaging and interactive learning journey**, encouraging them to share the experience with their sons and daughters, grandchildren, friends, and students. Join us on this educational adventure.

3. OBJECTIVES

The main purpose of this book, paired with the manual, is to offer education and awareness for children along with their families and teachers so that they acquire the tools to:

1. Live a life of physical and mental well-being.

2. Prevent the risk of developing diseases both in the present and in adulthood, such as diabetes, obesity, cardiovascular diseases, cancer, etc.

3. Spread important values for living within an inclusive and sustainable society, not only related to health, but also socially, to family and friendship ties, personal satisfaction, active participation in community life, and contributing to the community and the environment ("Give Back"), as taught by the centenarians of the Blue Zones (see paragraph 6.9 of this manual to further understand the Blue Zones and their characteristics).

4. Offer practical and achievable advice to start a healthy longevity and physical exercise journey immediately.

5. Create a "culture of longevity" based on health, well-being, positivity, personal sustainability, community, and environmental sustainability, as well as inclusion and solidarity.

4. USE

1. **Content and Adult Accompaniment:** Each page of the coloring book is full of useful and inspiring illustrations to explore the world of food, healthy nutrition, and exercise. These pages serve as conversation starters, prompting questions to engage children in discussions. Adults can act as guides, facilitating engaging learning and preparing for this task with the materials provided in the manual.

2. **Informative Content for Adults, Teachers, and Families:** The manual offers a series of informative texts for adults, teachers, and families to prepare for the educational moments with the children both at home and at school.

3. **Games and Practical Activities:** The book and in particular the manual also offer games and practical activities, making learning a fun and interactive experience. These activities can be carried out in the classroom so as to integrate the book into study programs and also at home and in the family environment.

4. **Healthy and Tasty Foods and Menus:** The book and manual include information on foods and simple and healthy menus and recipes, designed to involve children in choosing and preparing tasty and nutritious meals. Some cold recipes, which do not require cooking, are suitable for children and allow them to experiment in the kitchen, discovering healthy ingredients.

5. **Importance of Physical Activity:** We promote physical activity through fun exercises and practices that stimulate body movement, recognizing the importance of a healthy lifestyle from a young age. You will find some practical activities in the manual.

6. **Collaboration and Sharing of Family Tasks:** Through games and activities, we encourage collaboration within the family unit and teach children the importance of sharing household responsibilities equally.

7. **Learning English/Italian:** The book encourages learning English or Italian through simple words and sentences, allowing children, as well as adults, to become familiar with everyday terms.

8. **Methodology and Subjects Involved:** This book stimulates creativity, attention, and the expansion of children's knowledge in different areas such as geography, science, physical education, English/Italian, and art.

5. METHODOLOGY

We have created a series of illustrations to color in and interactive games to make learning an interesting and fun experience for children. They are designed to be used both at school and at home, involving teachers, families, and friends.

This is an approach based on edutainment (education + entertainment). Children become the protagonists, engaging in activities (always in pairs or groups to enhance collaboration, teamwork, and cohesion), such as:

a. **Storytelling** that leads to personal re-elaboration of concepts and their verbalization thanks to their creativity being stimulated.

b. **Role-Playing**, i.e., the simulation of real situations to create greater involvement and provide tools to learn and think both theoretically and practically.

c. **Group games** to create a moment of sharing in order to learn important concepts in a playful manner and absorb them better through cooperation.

d. **Problem Solving,** i.e., solving a problem to refine students' analytical and critical spirit and make them proactive and bearers of a solution and change, fully involving them in the situation that requires solving.

e. **Sharing circle.** Students sit in a circle with a facilitator (the teacher), who takes part in the circle. It is a space that allows participants to look each other in the eye, and there is no hierarchy, no beginning, or end. Many activities conclude with a moment of sharing, questions, and constructive debate to analyze and let what has been learned to settle and apply it in everyday life.

Each activity can be modified and adapted according to the teacher's needs, the type of students, and the time available. The guidelines are only general suggestions.

6. LEARNING GAMES

Let's Play Together at Home, at School, and With Friends!

1. The Mime Game: "What Food and in What Category?"

   a. You are divided into two teams and decide on the team name (a food).
   b. You have to take turns mimicking 1 food with proteins, 1 with fats, 1 with carbohydrates, 1 with fiber, 1 with vitamins, and 1 with minerals. The others have to guess.
   c. 1 group decides the food to mimic and how to mimic it.
   d. 1 team mimes and the opposite team has to guess.
   e. The teams take turns miming.
   f. The team that guesses the most wins.
   g. Final applause.

2. Guessing Game: "Guess What It Is?"

   a. Divide into two teams.
   b. Place different foods in bowls (vegetables, cereals, etc.).
   c. The two teams have to guess which foods they are and which category they belong to (carbohydrates, fats, proteins, fiber, vitamins, and minerals).
   d. The team that guesses the most wins.
   e. Final applause.

3. Mystery Test: "Let's Guess Blindfolded"

   a. Divide into two teams.
   b. Place different foods in bowls (vegetables, cereals, etc.)
   c. The participants are blindfolded, and the two teams have to guess which foods they are.
   d. When they try/touch food, in addition to guessing, they must indicate their sensations (smell, touch, taste, whether they like it or not).
   e. Final applause.

4. Recipe to Compose

a. Divide into two teams.
b. The 2 groups are given the same recipe on small sheets of paper, with a piece of paper for each ingredient and a piece of paper for each preparation step.
c. Prepare 2 posters and the 2 teams must put the ingredients and instructions in the right order.
d. At home, children can prepare the recipe with family or friends.
e. Final applause.
f. If you want, after the game you can prepare the recipes at home and invite friends to share the dish with you.

** For the recipes to compose, go to paragraph 8.1 of this manual, and for further recipes consult the booklet "Recipes and Menus" from the "Nutrition, Health, and Longevity" series and "At Longevity's Table" by The Valter Longo Foundation.*

The author's proceeds go to research and non-profit projects promoted by the Foundation itself, which aim to promote nutrition education in schools and provide nutritional assistance to people in particularly critical financial and health situations.

5. Role Playing. Let's Improvise!
At the Restaurant! (For Older Children)

a. Let's all become actors and act!
b. The restaurant game. All together we create a scene in the restaurant. 1 or 2 children are the owner/s, 3 or 4 (depending on the number of players) are the waiters/waitresses, 3 or 4 are the chefs/cooks, and the rest are the customers.
c. The restaurant does not have a healthy and good menu (you decide the restaurant menu together).
d. Create a dialogue with the owner, the chefs, the waiters, and the customers (the teacher moderates, and each pair of customers takes turns starting the dialogue with the staff).

e. Some customers argue with the owner, waiters, and chefs because the restaurant menu is unhealthy and, in turn, they try to defend the menu choice. Everyone tries to explain why they are right.

f. They propose changes to the menu, accepted by everyone.

g. As always, final applause.

6. Role Playing. Let's Improvise! Let's Invite Our Friends Over to Eat at Home! (For Older Children)

a. Let's all become actors and act!

b. We want to invite friends to our house for a special lunch or dinner.

c. Choose a special occasion (a birthday, end of school, etc.).

d. Together, create a healthy and delicious menu for your guests.

e. Also, explain why you think the menu is healthy.

f. The teacher or a family member moderates the discussion.

g. The same game can be played in other places: in a cooking school to become a chef and you discuss it with the teacher.

h. As always, final applause.

i. If you want, after the game you can prepare the menu at home with your family and invite friends to share a meal with you.

7. Food Movement (At School, at Home, With Friends)

a. Everyone moves slowly around the room in no particular order and the teacher or a family member moderates.

b. You choose one nutrient in turn (carbohydrates, proteins, fats, vitamins, and minerals). For example, carbohydrates.

c. The teacher or moderator, while the children keep moving around, says the names of foods, and if they contain carbohydrates everyone continues to move. If they don't contain them, they must stop.

Whoever doesn't stop leaves the game. We continue until 1 or 2 children (co-winners) remain.
d. Final applause.

8. The Food Dance (At School, at Home, With Friends)

a. Everyone moves in no particular order around the room and the teacher or a person from the family moderates or the children take turns.
b. Everyone chooses a food (carrot, potato, bread, water, etc.)
c. You choose a song to dance to.
d. At the start, everyone dances as they think their chosen food (carrot, potatoes, etc.) would dance for 5 -8 minutes.
e. Stop and sit in a circle and in pairs the children dance, and the others have to guess what food they are.
f. Final applause.

9. The Food Circle (At School)

a. Everyone sits on the floor or on chairs in a circle and the teacher moderates.
b. Everyone chooses one nutrient in turn (carbohydrates, proteins, fats, vitamins, and minerals).
c. In a circle in a clockwise direction, one after the other all the foods with a nutrient must be listed, for example carbohydrates.
d. Anyone who does not indicate the correct food must take a step back and leave the circle.
e. We continue until 1 or 2 children (co-winners) remain.
f. Final applause.

10. Let's Paint Good Foods

a. Create a drawing for your bedroom with all the foods you like and that help you grow! Hang it wherever you like!
b. As a class, create a display of drawings of your favorite foods.
c. Paint a paper plate with everything that you think is delicious, healthy, and tasty.

11. Let's Cook Together!

a.   Prepare a snack for school or an afternoon with friends.
b.   Let's cook together as a family!
c.   Enjoy your meal!

For snack recipes, go to paragraph 8.2 of this manual, and for further recipes and nutritional information see. the book "Longevity Begins as Children" by Professor Valter Longo (forthcoming in English) or "At Longevity's Table" by the Valter Longo Foundation.

The authors' proceeds go to research and non-profit projects promoted by the Foundation itself, which aim to promote nutrition education in schools and provide nutritional assistance to people in particularly critical financial and health situations.

7. INFORMATIVE MATERIALS FOR ADULTS, TEACHERS, FAMILIES

Introduction

In 2015, the United Nations approved the 2020 Agenda with 17 Sustainable Development Goals, among which is Objective 3 "Health and Well-being". Even before the pandemic **the increasing unpopularity of healthy eating and a balanced lifestyle** already represented a **real emergency** for high-income countries, while low-income countries have long been fighting against hunger and malnutrition. This situation of emergency, created in recent years following the spread of COVID-19, has highlighted how a healthy lifestyle and proper eating habits are essential not only to prevent the onset of numerous non-communicable diseases (cancer, diabetes, obesity, cardiovascular, autoimmune diseases such as multiple sclerosis, and neurodegenerative diseases such as Alzheimer's), but also to develop adequate immune resistance to external pathogens. For this reason, we will analyze important factors such as **healthy eating and exercise.** These are fundamental elements for our health that can also have a strong **environmental impact.** Finally, we will examine the Blue Zones, areas of the world where populations with numerous centenarians live, as an example of lifestyles for healthy longevity.

**** For more detailed information and in-depth analysis, please refer to Prof. Valter Longo's book "Longevity Begins as Children" (Milan: Vallardi, 2019) - Forthcoming in English*

[The author's proceeds are donated to research and non-profit projects]

7.1. THE CURRENT SITUATION: STARTING DATA AND ISSUES

7.1.1. The Modern and Postmodern World, Poor Knowledge and Attention Towards Food, and The Rise of Non-Communicable Diseases

The food we consume has significant consequences on fundamental aspects of our lives, such as our **physical and mental well-being, the quality of sleep, and the likelihood of non-communicable diseases,** which cannot be transmitted from one person to another (such as cancer, diabetes, obesity, cardiovascular, autoimmune, and neurodegenerative diseases). The relevance of nutrition as a fundamental element for our well-being is often neglected or poorly understood. The situation is made worse in high-income countries, by the **spread in the modern and postmodern world of** 1) **abundance and greater economic resources**, leading to increased consumption of many types of foods (e.g., meat) which affects health, and 2) **increasingly frenzied lifestyles** characterized by fast-paced rhythms, with little time and space to reflect on what foods are consumed every day and what the consequences are.

Another problem is the **spread of unhealthy dietary regimens**, such as consuming large quantities of sugars and starches, a trend that has spread to many countries, such as the United States and the Mediterranean area, due to a misinterpretation and reinterpretation of the healthy and traditional Mediterranean Diet in the countries where it originated.

This has led to a truly excessive consumption of bread, pasta, pizza, potatoes, as well as proteins. These foods are important for growth and energy intake, but they should not be eaten in excess, to avoid overweight and obesity or in deficit, to avoid malnutrition, both of which are the basis of many non-communicable diseases. The traditional Mediterranean Diet should act as a reference point, returning to eating as our ancestors did in the Mediterranean area (if you are Mediterranean), as well as a lifestyle in which physical exercise plays an important role. If you are not from the Mediterranean, the point of reference should be the healthy diet and food of your own ancestors, guided by information from the 5 pillars of longevity (see paragraph 7.6 for more information).

Poor attention and knowledge regarding what to eat and in what quantities, combined with the other problems described, have therefore contributed to generating a rather critical phase for public health, both present and future, both globally and in Italy. In fact, **in high-income countries, incorrect nutrition, and unbalanced lifestyles** (which result in **accelerated aging and excess weight**) have led to a real **epidemic of obesity and overweight**, which are at the root of the onset of **many non-communicable diseases.**

7.1.2. Obesity and Overweight: A Real Epidemic

It is estimated that today about 50% of adults and 30% of children and adolescents worldwide are overweight or obese. According to data from the **World Health Organization**, in 2016 about 1.9 million adults over the age of 18 were overweight, including 650 million obese people. The situation is no better among children and adolescents, with 340 million children or adolescents between the ages of 5 and 19 suffering from overweight or obesity in the same year. For example, if we look at the situation in Italy before the pandemic, the latest report on overweight and obesity (Italian Obesity Barometer Report 2019 - IBDO Foundation data in collaboration with ISTAT) indicates that **almost half of Italians are overweight and 1 out of every 10 is obese, and about 4 children or adolescents out of 10 are overweight or obese**, a percentage comparable to that of the United States of America.

It is a proven fact that overweight and obesity, scientifically defined as a disease, are risk factors for many non-communicable diseases (such as cancer, diabetes, cardiovascular diseases, autoimmune diseases such as multiple sclerosis, and neurodegenerative diseases such as Alzheimer's) both during childhood and adolescence and in adulthood. **The early years of life create the conditions for long a healthy life**. For example, **an obese child has a four times greater chance of developing adult-onset diabetes compared to a child of normal weight.** In addition, **excess weight during early life can predispose to developing or**

exacerbating conditions such as high blood pressure, hyperglycemia (pre-diabetes and type 2 diabetes), **liver diseases related to excess fat** (already very present in children), **gastrointestinal disorders** (constipation, gastroesophageal reflux, abdominal pain, and gallstones), **respiratory disorders** (bronchial asthma and sleep respiratory disorders), etc. Overweight and obesity also play a role in the onset of **multiple sclerosis and cardiovascular diseases** in children and adolescents (Brent Richard et al., *"Neurology"*, 2019).

Obesity and other diseases have also led and lead to a **high risk of mortality from COVID-19**. Obesity, in fact, has acquired an even greater importance following the COVID-19 emergency, which highlighted a significant increase in the risk of hospitalization and mortality among subjects suffering from this condition. According to ISTAT (The Italian National Institute of Statistics), overweight and obesity were strongly correlated with hospital admissions related to COVID-19, with a frequency double that of hospitalizations without mention of the virus. Furthermore, obesity, although rarely indicated as a direct cause of death, has been found to be a contributing factor in 4% of deaths among people who tested positive for the SARS-CoV-2 virus and in as many as 20% of deaths in individuals under the age of 49.

7.1.3. Excessively Sedentary and Inactive Behavior

In order to live a long and healthy life, it is essential not only to follow a balanced diet but also to **stay active and engage in physical activity every day**, a practice that should start in childhood and continue throughout adulthood and into the later stages of life. Unfortunately, this is not the norm for many young people, who lead a sedentary and inactive lifestyle: **more than 80% of adolescents do not engage in at least one hour of physical activity per day**, the minimum amount recommended by the World Health Organization (WHO, 2022). The lack of movement and time spent outdoors and in contact with nature are at the root of not only physical problems, but also mental issues such as stress, anxiety, and depression. This topic will be discussed in detail later.

7.1.4. The Effects of the Pandemic and Lockdown

The *lockdown* and pandemic have exacerbated and worsened many of the factors that negatively impact individual health and well-being, especially for young people. The first obstacle that young people had to deal with was the **limitation of in-person activities in schools,** which resulted in reduced opportunities to learn and grow and had **negative repercussions on their physical and mental health**. Other difficulties arose in relation to eating habits, the possibility of exercising, and the relationship with one's body. We will use Italy, a coutry critically hit by the pandemic, as a case study to analyze this situation.

1. **A survey conducted in Italy by OERSA (Observatory on Surplus, Recovery, and Food Waste) at CREA (Center for Food and Nutrition Research) has investigated how dietary habits have changed during an extraordinary period such as the first *lockdown*,** using a sample of 2900 people, each one belonging to a household, of which 22% have children under the age of 12. Respondents stated that they have increased their consumption of healthy foods: vegetables (33%), fruit (29%), legumes (26.5%), water (22%), and extra virgin olive oil (21.5%). However, 44.5% admitted to having eaten more sweets and 16% to having drunk more wine. Also, **44% of respondents gained weight due to a higher caloric intake and less physical activity, which affected 53% of the sample.** Consequently, over 37% of cases expressed the need to go on a diet. According to a report by the organization Save the Children dated April 2020, almost half of Italian families (44.7%) **have had to change their dietary habits during the pandemic due to reduced financial availability,** which often limited access to quality raw ingredients and forced unbalanced nutrition.

2. Children and adolescents have been deprived of most of the social, recreational, and sports activities that play a central role in their growth and development. In particular, a study coordinated by the University of Pisa (Fornili et al, PLOS ONE, 2021) highlighted a **correlation between the reduction in opportunities to engage in physical activity and the onset**

of severe symptoms of anxiety and depression, concluding that maintaining the same levels of physical activity during lockdown would have reduced the number of severe cases of anxiety or depression in the population by 21%.

3. Children forced to stay inside their homes have had to deal with an **increasingly conflicting relationship with food and their bodies.** The phenomena of anorexia, bulimia, and binge eating disorder have been exacerbated and worsened by the pandemic, particularly among **minors and young girls,** and the onset age of eating disorders has progressively decreased, moving from high school years to middle school. These are the findings published in March 2021 by ADI ONLUS, the Italian Association of Dietetics and Clinical Nutrition. In a press release, the association reports that **the pandemic has not only worsened pre-existing cases but has also coincided with a 30% increase in new diagnoses,** even among the youngest, and requests for hospitalization among minors under the age of 14. Many students have reported episodes of emotional hunger caused by boredom, stress, and constant access to food, and the inability to relieve stress with extracurricular activities and socialization has led many young people to focus on goals related to aesthetic appearance, often through unhealthy eating behaviors.

4. An IPSOS survey conducted in 2021 in collaboration with the Spallanzani National Institute for Infectious Diseases, the Gemelli Polyclinic in Rome, Italy, and the Pediatric Hospital Bambino Gesù showed that more than one in three children and **43% of teenagers have experienced weight gain during the pandemic,** which is even more alarming considering that Italy was already in fourth place in Europe for the percentage of obese children (9.4%) and overweight children (20.4%) (IPSOS, 2021).

7.1.5. Lifestyle and Environmental Issues

In addition to being unhealthy and not promoting longevity, many habits (both dietary and non-dietary) adopted by a substantial portion of the population are **harmful to the environment.** Examples include massive consumption of meat and motorized transportation. Moreover, many of the mechanisms that regulate **food production and consumption processes are not environmentally sustainable.** Among the main problems related to food systems are **global warming** due to **greenhouse gas emissions, erosion, deforestation,** and **reduction of biodiversity, as well as intensive exploitation of water resources.** The significant **food waste** that occurs in high-income countries also has a strongly negative impact on the environment. This topic will be discussed in detail later.

7.2. SOLUTIONS: BALANCED DIET AND PHYSICAL EXERCISE

Among the factors to never lose sight of in order to maintain health and prevent the onset of non-communicable diseases, there are certainly a **healthy and balanced diet and physical exercise.** Recognized scientific studies demonstrate that in some cases, diseases such as diabetes, various types of cancer, and cardiovascular diseases could be easily countered through **useful and fundamental modifications to nutrition and lifestyle, focused on healthy longevity.** If we focus on Italy's specific case, for example, **over a third of diseases or premature deaths could be avoided.** Therefore, these are significant percentages: 36.9% of men and 18.5% of women die before the age of 75 due to avoidable factors. The largest cause of this type of death is represented by cancers (43.8%), particularly lung cancer (34.7%); followed by cardiovascular diseases, entirely represented by ischemic heart diseases (31.9%) (data from the Ialian Ministry of Health).

The benefits that come from adopting a balanced diet and a healthy lifestyle, however, are not limited to individual benefits. **Preventing diseases through taking care of one's lifestyle can not only save many lives** and allow a significant number of people to live better and longer, **but it is also necessary for nations and states at a global level,** through the reduction of public spending. With regard to Italian national healthcare spending, for example, it is estimated that **cardiovascular diseases cost the Italian state approximately 21 billion euros each year** (NSIS, New Healthcare Information System), **cancer costs 19 billion euros** (AIOM, Italian

Association of Medical Oncology), **and diabetes 12 billion euros** (IDF Diabetes Atlas, International Diabetes Federation - Diabetes Atlas).

To promote a lifestyle that lays the foundation for a healthy and long life, it is, therefore, important to **educate and raise awareness amongst the population regarding healthy longevity and the importance of nutrition and lifestyle,** as well as other factors related to longevity such as socialization, sense of family, friendships, purpose in life, solidarity, and inclusion. These values are essential for living a long and healthy life, as proven by the centenarians of the Blue Zones, the regions in the world with record longevity (Ikaria in Greece, Nicoya in Costa Rica, Okinawa in Japan, Loma Linda in California, and Ogliastra in Sardinia, Italy).

These issues must also be addressed, especially with children and young people, emphasizing their importance in improving the quality of life from a young age, whilst **countering false myths and widespread misinformation,** teaching them to **distinguish and recognize qualified and reliable sources of information.**

A separate discussion must be reserved for the **solutions that need to be adopted to limit the climate crisis,** as urgent as the health crisis. In particular, the **transformation and streamlining of the food systems** as we know them today and the **choice of a predominantly plant-based diet** are necessary elements for the safeguarding of human health and the planet for future generations.

7.3. STRATEGY 1: UNDERSTAND THAT WE ARE WHAT WE EAT

The main reason for following a healthy diet is **to live well, energetically, long, and in good health.** We are what we eat: the type of food we consume and when we do it can have a **decisive influence on our well-being, on the duration and quality of sleep, fertility, and the likelihood of developing a tumor. Not only our physical health but also our mental health** depends upon what we eat. Everything we eat, even seemingly healthy foods like chicken meat, can be harmful if, for example, associated with high daily protein consumption or if it contains hormones or antibiotics.

What a newborn, child, and teenager eat conditions the way and speed with which every organ of their body forms and functions for decades, if not for their entire life. For example, consuming too much protein in a child is associated with a high risk of several diseases; on the other hand, a diet with insufficient protein levels can cause growth and malnutrition problems. The result is visible in their physical appearance in terms of height, obesity or thinness, and more or less developed muscle mass. Additionally, the effects are visible in terms of health; such as children who tend to get sick frequently or have learning difficulties at school.

The diet we follow is **the most important and easily controllable factor for us,** in addition to physical exercise. It is essential to consider that many components of our diet are not just foods, but also **powerful molecules capable of determining significant changes in our bodies, and it is important to understand what they are and how they work.**

Proteins

Proteins are one of the three main macronutrients, along with carbohydrates and fats. They are important because **they provide the necessary elements for the creation and functioning of cells.** However, an excess of proteins can be harmful. The structural component of proteins is amino acids, which are important namely for their structural function since they form all tissues in our body. In particular moments of life, such as pregnancy, early childhood, and growth, this process is particularly important for the development of new tissues or for the conservation of existing tissues. However, for most of our adult life, the quantity of protein physically required by your body is roughly 0.8 grams of protein per kg (0.36 grams per pound) of body weight, so a smaller amount than that should be normally consumed.

Meat is a well-known source of protein, but it is not healthy if consumed in excess. It is certainly necessary **to eliminate processed meats,** classified by the World Health Organization as "type 1 carcinogens", such as sausages, and smoked or canned meats. It is also important to **be careful with red meats,** indicated instead as "type 2 carcinogens", which are a possible cause of cancer. On the other hand, it is essential to **maximize the consumption of plant-based proteins** (such as those found in legumes), including fish occasionally, and, for older adults, limited amounts of animal-based proteins in order to avoid the risk of malnutrition. If lactose sensitivity is not a problem, it is also possible to consume dairy products, but not in too much excess, provided they come from animals that graze freely and are not given hormones or high doses of antibiotics. Goat dairy products are preferable.

Carbohydrates

Carbohydrates are our **main source of energy** and are found in most of the foods we eat, in the form of simple carbohydrates, such as the sugar contained in fruit juices, honey, sweets, or sugary drinks, or in a complex form, such as the large chains of glucose and other sugars contained in vegetables or whole grains **also in the form of starches.**

As a general rule, **the caloric intake of carbohydrates (vegetables included) should cover 45%-60% of the daily energy requirement.** The intake of 4 servings of carbohydrates during the day is recommended, for example, 2 servings of pasta or rice (not too much and preferably "al dente"), plus 2 servings of bread. Furthermore, according to the World Health Organization, consuming between one and a half to three servings of whole grains, preferably organic, would have the advantage of providing more fiber and vitamins and reducing the risk of chronic diseases such as type 2 diabetes, obesity, and hypertension.

Fats

Lipids or fats are **the main source of stored energy in the human body.** In addition to this role, modified fat molecules **play a fundamental role in many structures and functions of the cells of the entire organism.** In particular, they have a central function in the formation of cell membranes and hormones. Fats can be **saturated** (such as those found in butter) **or unsaturated.** Unsaturated fats are further divided into monounsaturated (such as oleic acid found in olive oil) and polyunsaturated (such as those found in salmon and corn oil seeds). Omega-3 and omega-6 polyunsaturated fats are called "essential fatty acids" because the human body cannot produce them, but they are essential for its proper functioning.

On the other hand, the consumption of unsaturated and trans fats (that have been subjected to chemical modification and are found, for example, in foods such as margarine, packaged sweets, fillings and cake glazes, pizza, cookies, fast food, etc.) can lead to the development of diabetes and cardiovascular disease in adulthood.

Fat intake within a diet is very important, however, it would be advisable to **prefer foods rich in unsaturated fats, especially extra-virgin olive oil, fish, and nuts.**

Micronutrients

Micronutrients, namely vitamins and minerals, are **important for biochemical reactions,** enzymes, hormones, and other substances necessary for the development and proper functioning of our body's "machine." For example, vitamin D (found in salmon, canned sardines, herring, etc.), zinc (found in sesame seeds, pumpkin seeds, etc.), and iron (in clams, mussels, lentils, coconut, etc.) are important for the immune system, while calcium (found in sheep and goat milk or partially skimmed cow's milk, low-fat yogurt, shrimp, etc.) and vitamin D help maintain normal bone mineral density.

Although **a diet rich in vegetables, fish, nuts (walnuts, almonds, hazelnuts, etc.), and whole grains** is the best way to obtain essential nutrients, even highly nutritious diets can be deficient in vitamin D and, in the case of vegans and older adults, vitamin B12. In addition, few people in the world consume a highly nutritious diet that supplies all the aforementioned deficiencies. For this reason, a dietician or pediatrician can help understand if there are deficiencies and know the appropriate supplementation in the specific case.

7.4. STRATEGY 2: KNOW THE MEDITERRANEAN DIET, ITS IMPORTANCE, AND ITS ISSUES

The eating habits of Italians have long been the focus of scholars. The **American biologist and epidemiologist Ancel Keys** arrived **in the Cilento area,** in the province of Salerno near Naples in Southern Italy, at the beginning of the 1950s to study a **population that seemed protected from heart diseases and had low cholesterol levels.** He observed that the most common meal consisted of a vegetable soup or "minestrone", pasta always served with tomato and a bit of cheese (and, only occasionally, small pieces of meat or fish), a large amount of fresh vegetables, red wine, and fresh fruit.

Thus, the myth of the Mediterranean Diet was born, a healthy and longevity-promoting diet that unites a very diverse region made up of Mediterranean countries such as Greece, Italy, Spain, Turkey, Cyprus, Morocco, etc. It is a diet characterized by rich and ancient traditions, and products coming from different continents, such as eggplant from Persia and tomatoes from the Americas. In these geographical areas, the common denominator in terms of food is the presence of **legumes, cereals (mostly whole grains), dried fruits, vegetables in large quantities and preferably in season, fish, and extra virgin olive oil.** Red meat, on the other hand, is part of the foods to be consumed in moderation, together with dairy products. However, the Mediterranean Diet is much more than a mere list of foods. It is instead a lifestyle based on a cultural identity made of **creativity, dialogue, hospitality, respect for the land, and biodiversity, which has a strongly positive impact on health.**

However, with the myth of the Mediterranean Diet, there has also been a tendency, encouraged by Keys himself, to **consume large quantities of sugars and starches,** such as those found in pasta and bread, and **to demonize fats.** This is an incorrect interpretation of this dietary regime. These "misinterpreted" eating habits have contributed to the world's largest **epidemic of obesity and metabolic diseases in the US and elsewhere.** In fact, currently, **almost 25% of the world's population suffers from metabolic syndrome,** which is a set of risk factors such as excess body fat, high levels of "bad" LDL cholesterol and triglycerides in the blood, and high blood pressure, and is therefore at risk of developing diabetes and cardiovascular diseases, etc. Furthermore, it must be recognized that the Mediterranean Diet, traditionally consumed by the centenarians In Italy, **has now been abandoned by most Italians,** who consume milk, cheese, white meat, and red meat much more frequently, thus more closely approaching the modern diet followed by populations in the United States and Northern Europe.

The traditional Mediterranean diet is the reference point to follow. Nevertheless, we have to remember again that individuals who are not from the Mediterranean should look to the healthy diet and food of their own ancestors, guided by information from the 5 pillars of longevity. Some individual foods, taken separately, are healthy, but in our world, they are consumed excessively by both children and adults. For example, Italians eat **an excess of bread, pasta, pizza, potatoes, and proteins.** This corresponds to ten tablespoons of sugar every day. These foods should not be eliminated, but excess consumption, as with anything, creates problems as well as deficiencies. The mistake of completely or almost completely eliminating carbohydrates from the diet, enticed by rapid weight loss, can turn into a health hazard. In adults, this is associated with a reduction in longevity and an increase in diseases. Therefore, it is also not recommended for children and teenagers. These foods should be consumed moderately. In addition, there is **excess consumption of proteins and red meats, low consumption of grains and legumes, and a lack of variety in vegetables** that have characterized the diet of most Italians since the 1960s and other countries in the world. Excess (and this cannot be stressed enough) is therefore what needs to be highlighted, not elimination. Being mindful of not overdoing it is essential for balance and good health.

The Mediterranean Diet is, therefore, healthy **"only if followed as grandparents did.** They ate **little pasta,** lightly seasoned, with **green beans and less bread.** They used to eat plenty of soups, made with the "poor" products of the land, because there was no money for anything else. In this case, yes, it does pay off. Even more so if combined with constant physical activity. At the moment, for example, only 10% of Italian families really follow it. There is enormous room for improvement. Without a change of course, Italy will inevitably be a seriously ill country. Even for Covid, it was precisely the obese, people with age-relatd diseases, and older adults who were by far the most prone." (Valter Longo, Valter Longo Foundation Onlus - Redazione. "Valter Longo: The Mediterranean Diet Has Been Distorted, Followed Like This It's Harmful." November 18, 2020).

As a result, the changes, speed, and abundance related to the lifestyle in the modern and postmodern world, far from the ancient reality of the Mediterranean world that gave birth to the famous diet, have led to excess, particularly in terms of quantity. For this reason, it is necessary to revisit the Mediterranean Diet based on these transformations that have taken place in our world and develop more precise and complex diets that promote longevity in good health, in order to offer more detailed information in the confusion that we often find ourselves navigating with regards to nutrition.

7.5. STRATEGY 3: FOLLOW A DIET THAT PROMOTES LONGEVITY AND HEALTH FOR CHILDREN

These guidelines take into account clinical, epidemiological, and basic research studies carried out by Professor Longo's team in Italian and international research centers, as well as the dietary habits of centenarians and children from populations with longevity records. They also correspond to international and Italian guidelines for the diet of children and young people (LARN, Reference Intake Levels of Nutrients and Energy for the Italian Population 2014; WHO, World Health Organization; WCRF, World Cancer Research Fund).

Before sharing a series of tips, it is essential to remember that food is also a pleasure and changing one's dietary system should not be so challenging as to lead those who had decided to change it to give up. For this reason, the preference was not to revolutionize eating habits but rather to attempt to limit the changes to only include the truly significant ones.

1. The Longevity Diet for children and adolescents is complete and includes all nutrients: plant and animal proteins, carbohydrates, and fats. It should be noted that there is a percentage of underweight children. Many of the rules described here apply to them, but others do not, as they may lose further weight. It is therefore important for them to increase the amount of starch consumed.

2. Regulate the amount of protein according to age. Children and adolescents should consume the following grams of protein per kilogram of body weight per day: 0.9 grams per kg (0.4 g per pound) from 4 years and up.

    For example, a 9-month-old child weighing 9 kg (19.8 lb.) should consume 11.7 g of protein per kg (5.3 g per lb.), a 3-year-old child weighing 14 kg (30.8 lb.) should consume 14 g per kg (5.3 g per lb.), and a 10-year-old child weighing 30 kg (66 lb.) should consume approximately 27 g per day per kg (13 g per lb.). It is important to understand that too little protein can lead to malnutrition and slow growth, but too much can cause a variety of other problems.

3. Introduce both plant-based proteins from legumes and nuts, and animal-based proteins from fish (2-3 times a week, avoiding those with high mercury content) and less frequently consume red meat, white meat, and eggs (one portion per week for each of these foods, preferably organic).

4. Consume abundant quantities of low glycemic index carbohydrates (legumes, vegetables), decreasing foods that are too rich in starch (pasta, bread, pizza, potatoes, and rice) and sugars (fruit, fruit juices, snacks, and sugary carbonated drinks). Note: limiting does not mean avoiding, therefore the right amounts can be consumed by minimizing snacks and sugary drinks. The mistake of completely or almost completely eliminating carbohydrates from the diet, enticed by rapid weight loss, can turn into health damage. In adults, this is associated with reduced longevity and increased disease risk. Therefore, it is also not recommended for children and teenagers.

5. Be careful with whole grains and foods that are too rich in fiber such as legumes, if the child or teenager starts to have intestinal problems. Consult a pediatric gastroenterologist if necessary.

6. Minimize saturated, hydrogenated, and trans fats. Limit salt and sugar, although an occasional sweet treat is fine, especially those that are a bit healthier, based on fruit or dark chocolate.

7. Eat within a 12-hour window, have dinner not too late, by 8 pm, avoid nighttime snacks, and have breakfast around 8 am. This is important, especially for overweight and obese children and teenagers. It is, in fact, widely documented, particularly in adults, that, with the same calorie intake, those who consume meals within 11-12 hours have a lower risk of overweight and cardiovascular diseases. These effects are due to an optimization of the sleep-wake rhythm, which in turn improves our metabolism. If children/teenagers wake up early, breakfast can be postponed as much as possible to maintain their eating window. For example, if they finish dinner at 8:30 pm but wake up at 7 am, breakfast should be postponed as close to 8:30 am as possible. If this is a problem for school, then dinner should be earlier. Obviously, this is more important for overweight or potentially overweight children/teenagers. For others, extending the period in which they eat to 13 hours is fine.

8. Meals and snacks should be a maximum of 4-5 times a day.

9. Eat more, not less. For children in general, and especially for those who are overweight, replace some of the foods containing high amounts of starch, such as pasta, bread, rice, or potatoes, with vegetables and legumes, which are rich in fiber and therefore give a greater sense of satiety. For example, remove 50-60 grams (1.7-2 oz) of these foods every day and replace them with 100 gr (3.5 oz) or more grams of carrots, broccoli, chickpeas, beans, etc.

10. Do not exaggerate with the rules, but find the best strategy

for each case, possibly with the help of a nutritionist. For example, we can allow a can of soda and a pizza per week if it makes children and teenagers happy, and we can make the substitutions suggested in point 9 of this list.

11. Eat slowly and avoid the TV. It is good to eat slowly, with the TV off and phones away. Paying attention to what you eat helps to better achieve a sense of satiety, avoiding unnecessary calorie intake.

12. Eat by selecting the right healthy ingredients among those eaten by our ancestors, our parents, grandparents, and great-grandparents (for example, for Italians: olive oil, legumes, etc.) and preferably those from the local tradition, seasonal, and of organic origin, based on one's possibilities and availability. This helps to limit the consumption of fast food and industrially processed foods. In addition to this advantage, choosing the right ingredients among those present in the table of our ancestors could potentially protect us from the onset of intestinal and/or autoimmune diseases (intolerances, allergies, Crohn's disease, colitis, celiac disease, etc.). The mechanism is not yet clear, but consuming the wrong foods is often associated with increased inflammation and autoimmune diseases.

13. Exercise at least one hour and one hour of walking per day. For adults, guidelines vary.

For adults the guidelines differ.

Taken from "Longevity Begins as Children" (forthcoming in English) by Professor Valter Longo, where you will find more in-depth information as well as recipes and menus.

The author's proceeds go to research and non-profit projects promoted by the Valter Longo Foundation, which aim to promote nutrition education in schools and provide nutritional assistance to people in particularly critical financial and health situations.

7.6. STRATEGY 4: RECOGNIZE THE LEADING EXPERTS TO FOLLOW AND THE PILLARS OF THE STUDY OF HEALTHY LONGEVITY

Many people think they are nutrition experts and dispense advice or suggest diets without being nutritionists or doctors, without even knowing what it means to eat "the right amount". The experts to follow regarding nutrition are **doctors and researchers specialized in nutrition** (i.e. internists, biochemists, nutritionists, dieticians, etc.) who hold university positions and work in important institutions, and **experts in various fields of experimentation and study** (especially referring to the five pillars: basic research, epidemiological studies, clinical studies, studies on centenarians, and the study of complex systems described later), who participate in scientific research and clinical activities in the nutritional field. In this sense, the doctor, the nutritionist, and/or the dietitian can provide the right indications regarding who are the experts to refer to and how to practice an ad hoc diet, also in relation to any disease and the presence of food intolerances.

THE 5 PILLARS OF LONGEVITY RESEARCH

To navigate and extract the right information in terms of nutrition, Professor Valter Longo suggests focusing on five areas of study called the Pillars of Longevity, as many doctors and researchers around the world already do. Nutritional information received from experts can be considered truly reliable only if the experts have analyzed the results and information coming from these five areas/pillars as a basis for their observations: basic research, epidemiological studies on populations, clinical studies, studies on centenarians, and studies of complex systems. This process is very useful to understand how science proceeds, particularly in the field of nutrition, and who to refer to.

1. Basic Research and Juventology/Biogerontology

Juventology is the study of youth and "healthspan", or the period of life during which a person remains young and healthy. Starting from studies conducted on simple organisms (such as yeasts and cells), it is possible to understand the interaction between cells and nutrients, as well as how a certain type of diet can positively influence health and determine longevity. The results of these studies are then verified on humans. This is the first step to start with. In fact, starting from more or less simple organisms, it is then possible to translate these basic discoveries into valid strategies for humans.

2. Epidemiology (Population Studies)

Epidemiology refers to the frequency with which diseases occur and the factors that stimulate or hinder the development of diseases in different populations, testing the hypotheses of basic research. Through this discipline, by analyzing the frequency of certain diseases in a population and the diet commonly followed by it, hypotheses can be developed about how diet impacts metabolism and the likelihood of developing diseases.

3. Clinical Studies

In order to demonstrate that a diet impacts health, **clinical studies** are necessary. These are medical studies on people that test the effectiveness of hypotheses formulated from basic and epidemiological research. For example, one group of pre-diabetics is asked to maintain their current diet, while another group is asked to maintain their diet but reduce their sugar intake. The effects of the different diets are then compared between the two groups, and conclusions are drawn in support or not of the basic and epidemiological research.

It is important to note that clinical studies should adhere to Good Clinical Practice (GCP) standards, which are international ethical and scientific quality standards necessary for designing, conducting, registering, and reporting a clinical trial involving human subjects.

4. Study of Centenarians

Studies conducted on populations around the world with a high percentage of centenarians allow for concrete data on the effectiveness of certain dietary and lifestyle habits maintained throughout an entire life. Diet, together with a healthy and active lifestyle, exercise, socializing, and spirituality is the basis for a healthy and long life. The dietary and lifestyle habits of the healthiest groups of centenarians in various areas of the world are analyzed, especially those living in the famous Blue Zones characterized by longevity: Loma Linda in California, Nicoya in Costa Rica, Ikaria in Greece, Okinawa in Japan and Ogliastra (Sardinia) in Italy. These analyses offer data and a solid foundation regarding the safety, effectiveness, and acceptance of a particular dietary approach.

5. Study of Complex Systems

To understand the complexity of the human body, it is compared to a complex system such as a car or an airplane. For example, the interactions between food, damage, and aging in the human body are analyzed and compared to complex systems such as airplanes. This allows for a deeper and more simplified understanding of certain functions of the human body. Sugar, for instance, can be compared to gasoline for a car as a source of energy. If consumed in excess and in combination with certain types of fats (such as saturated fats), it activates aging genes, insulin resistance genes, and hyperglycemia genes, contributing directly and indirectly to the onset of diseases. Similarly, a car needs fats, such as oil for brakes and engines, and if they are of the wrong type or low quality, the engine wears out more quickly.

To understand the dietary indications that guarantee a healthy and long life, it is advisable to refer to these pillars. As evidence of this, let's examine the high-protein, high-fat, and low-carbohydrate diet, i.e., lots of meat and little bread, pasta, etc. Following the 5 pillars, we see how:

1. Laboratory studies indicate that high intake of protein and saturated fats is associated with mutations of cells and the entire organism that lead to accelerated aging and the onset of diseases;

2. Epidemiological and clinical studies show negative long-term effects;

3. Populations with record longevity do not follow it.

In conclusion, a high-protein, high-fat, and low-carbohydrate diet is based only on 1 or 2 pillars and therefore does not have all the necessary scientific evidence to indicate that it can optimize health and longevity.

Recommendations for a diet that guarantees a long and healthy life should be **based on solid and concrete evidence,** founded on basic, clinical, genetic, and epidemiological research, and thousands of patients followed directly. In addition, most dietary advice corresponds to the nutritional habits of populations characterized by good health and record longevity, where diet is a central factor. It is therefore recommended to keep this reference in mind when reading or receiving advice on nutrition and lifestyle, to understand in whom to place one's trust and health.

7.7. STRATEGY 5: BE AWARE OF THE IMPORTANCE OF PHYSICAL EXERCISE

The most influential **factor** in determining how long we live is **genetic:** we inherit modified genes from our ancestors that protect us against the risk of age-related diseases. However, inheritance alone is not enough. If we want to ensure a long and healthy life, there are at least two other factors we must take care of. The first is nutrition, which should be healthy and balanced, as already discussed. But if we want to have an edge in delaying the aging process and thus reducing the risk of disease, it is necessary to add another fundamental aspect to our lifestyle: **regularly and consistently practicing physical activity** every day throughout our lives. Researchers who have focused their attention on the analysis of **long-lived populations,** characterized by the presence of centenarians, have noticed how **constant physical activity,** even in **older age,** constitutes a common denominator, as well as a healthy diet.

If constant physical activity allows us to stay healthy until older age, **the lack of exercise is instead correlated with the onset of diseases** such as obesity and overweight, type 2 diabetes, cardiovascular diseases (caused by an increase in cholesterol, blood pressure, triglycerides, etc.), the risk of colon, uterine, breast, and lung cancer, reduced bone mass, and the risk of osteoporosis.

These problems negatively impact individuals' lives and weigh on public spending and healthcare spending.

Children and Teenagers, Often Too Sedentary, and the Benefits of Physical Exercise

A healthy diet and the practice of physical exercise are essential elements for the **development of the individual, starting from the early years of life.** When these elements are lacking, there are signs that we should learn to recognize in order to promptly address them, such as cavities, dermatitis, acne (especially between the ages of 11 and 17), anemia, and allergies (mainly to dairy products and eggs). It is therefore essential that even the youngest start taking care of their lifestyle and lay the foundations for a long and healthy life.

The **World Health Organization** recommends that preadolescents and adolescents engage in **at least one hour of moderate to intense physical activity per day,** depending on individual capabilities and circumstances. This includes not only individual or team sports, but also active transportation (such as walking or biking) and recreational activities both in and outside of school settings.

There are three concerning aspects to the data: **only a minority of adolescents engage in enough physical exercise, healthy daily physical activity habits decrease between the ages of 11 and 15, and the situation has worsened compared to past decades. More than 80% of adolescents do not reach the recommended daily activity threshold** (WHO, 2022). The situation is present in many countries. For example, a 2001 report from the Higher Institute of Health in Italy estimated that 86.7% of adolescents did not engage in the appropriate amount of physical activity, a percentage that rose to 90.6% when considering only girls. Comparing these statistics to those of 2016, the situation has worsened, with the respective percentages at 88.6% and 91.5%.

For children, the benefits of engaging in sports or physical activities go beyond physical well-being. Sports help **develop values and skills that can be applied in various contexts, such as the importance of commitment and perseverance to achieve good**

results, the organization required for **time management** between physical activity and academic obligations, the **ability to overcome obstacles and improve, collaboration, and team spirit.** Moreover, several studies, such as those by Professor John Ratey at Harvard Medical School (http://www.johnratey.com/), suggest that **physical exercise can prepare students' brains to learn, process, and optimally remember information.** The professor also suggests that physical activity increases stress resistance, allowing students to approach academic obligations with greater peace of mind.

General Guidelines for Physical Exercise

Often, it is sufficient to adopt some simple precautions or change some daily habits to adopt a more active lifestyle that allows for significant improvement in the quality of life of young people.

1. Walk, cycle, and **move outdoors for at least one hour a day.**

2. Do **bodyweight exercises,** using **weights** in alternate days, and **go for a walk on the weekend.**

3. **Maintain an "active lifestyle"** by getting used to taking the stairs, walking, or biking to school, and helping parents with household chores.

4. Avoid being sedentary and inactive: **limit the hours spent on the computer, tablet, and TV.**

5. **Pair studying with practicing a sport,** trying to coordinate school commitments with sports commitments. If this proves to be complicated, don't abandon sports but find a solution to continue pairing it with studying, such as reducing the duration of workouts or participating in fewer competitive events.

6. **Bone mass** can be "accumulated" thanks to sports that promote mineralization and the development of bone structure in children and adolescents. These include running, dancing, climbing, basketball, volleyball, and in general sports where one runs and jumps.

7. Consume **easily digestible meals with a low glycemic index, a few hours before practicing sports.** After sports, consume a source of **preferably whole grain carbohydrates** together with **lean and easily digestible sources of protein** (for example, a fish-based main course accompanied by a side of vegetables dressed with extra virgin olive oil, if available, and a slice of whole wheat bread).

8. If you stop practicing sports or reduce your hours of physical activity, adapt your diet to your new lifestyle: **if you move less, you need to ingest fewer calories.**

** Taken from "Longevity Begins as Children" (forthcoming in English) by Professor Valter Longo, where you will find more in-depth information as well as recipes and menus.*

The author's proceeds go to research and non-profit projects promoted by the Valter Longo Foundation itself, which aim to promote nutrition education in schools and provide nutritional assistance to people in particularly critical financial and health situations.

7.8. STRATEGY 6: BE AWARE OF THE IMPACT OF LIFESTYLE ON THE ENVIRONMENT

An element that should be central to the debate on environmental sustainability is the **transformation and efficiency of food systems** as we know them today, necessary for the safeguarding of human health and the planet for future generations. In particular, **the efficiency of food production and distribution systems is central to achieving many of the 17 Sustainable Development Goals** of the UN's 2030 Agenda, including SDG 2 **"Zero Hunger"**, SDG 3 **"Good Health and Well-being"**, SDG 12 **"Responsible Consumption and Production"**, SDG 13 **"Climate Action"**, SDG 14 **"Life Below Water"**, and SDG 15 **"Life on Land"**.

Global Changes Can Save the Earth

The **intensive exploitation of cultivable land** (which accounts for up to 72% of land) carried out to feed a growing demand for food (and unfortunately, massive waste), has allowed the world population to quadruple in a century (from 1.9 in 1920 to 7.7 billion in 2020), but with numerous negative consequences for the environment. Among these, **the increase in greenhouse gases due to deforestation, the decrease in biodiversity and erosion, and soil impoverishment** phenomena, up to the **desertification** of entire areas, stand out. These serious problems can be avoided using sustainable and non-intensive agronomic and zootechnical techniques. It should also be remembered that **most arable land, over 60% in Europe, is used for fodder production for livestock.** It is therefore urgent to reverse the processes of food production and consumption, to reduce CO_2 emissions by up to 6 billion tons per year.

The current food system (the entire supply chain, from food production to consumption) generates **around 30% of all human greenhouse gas emissions,** and it is leading to heat waves that have caused **temperatures to rise by as much as 1.2 °C (34.16 °F)** above pre-industrial levels. Experts sound the alarm: exceeding 1.5 °C (34.7 °F) would lead to even more serious climate disruptions than those currently experienced. Encouraging a change in food systems to save our planet and have a healthier population should therefore also be a political objective.

Although a global political intervention remains imperative to change the food industry, individually we can contribute by changing our eating habits. Diet is indeed an important element in saving the planet, as indicated in the **report produced by the *Eat-Lancet Commission on Food, Planet, and Health*** published in one of the world's leading medical journals, "Lancet". The report was produced in 2019 by 37 scientists from 16 countries to define **on rigorous scientific grounds some healthy ("Planetary Health Diets") diets for humans and the planet that are sustainable in terms of production and consumption of food.**

What does a healthy planetary diet mean? For example, limited or no consumption of meat, especially red meat, and dairy, a reduction in sugars, and, conversely, attention to nuts, vegetables, fruits, whole grains, plant proteins, and unsaturated fats that can have, as previously indicated, a positive impact on personal and environmental health. These general guidelines, as well as the flexibility and adaptability of diets, and respect for health and the environment, are elements that are **common to the *Longevity Diet and the Planetary Health Diet* outlined by "Lancet".** The IPCC (Intergovernmental Panel on Climate Change), the UN scientific committee, has also highlighted the need to shift the diet towards a plant-based food regime through the report **"Climate Change and Land"** disseminated in August 2019.

The following table compares the two diets in order to highlight their similarities and differences.

FOODS		PLANETARY DIET Ideal quantity per week (g/oz-lb)	LONGEVITY DIET Ideal quantity per week (g)
Red meat		0-100 g /0-3.5 oz	0 (before the age of 65)
White meat		0-400 g/0-14 oz	0 (before the age of 65)
Fish		0-700 g/0-1.5 lb.	200-300 g/7-10 oz
Dairy products		0-3500 g/0-7.7 lb.	0 (before the age of 65)
Eggs		0-175 g/0-6 oz	0-120 g/0-4.2 oz
Nuts		0-500 g/0-1 lb.	200-300/7-10 oz
Legumes		0-700 g/0-1.5 lb.	700-1700/1.5-3.7 lb.
Cereals		0-1600 g/0-3.5 lb.	700-2000/1.5-4.4 lb.
Potatoes		0-700 g/0-1.5 lb.	400-2800/0.8-6 lb.
Fruit		700-2100 g/1.5 -4.6 lb.	1050 g/2.3 lb.
Vegetables		1400-4200 g/3- 9.2 lb.	1400-3000/3-6.6 lb.
Unsaturated fats		140-560 g/5-19.7 oz	400-500/0.8-1 lb.
Saturated fats		0-83 g/0-3 oz	0-40 g/0-1.4 oz
Added sugars		0-217 g/0-7.6 oz	0-100 g/ 0-3.5 oz
Sources		**www.thelancet.com** **vol 393** **February 2, 2019**	**At Longevity's Table** **Valter Longo Foundation**

Food, Climate, and Health

One of the least sustainable elements of the current population's diet is certainly the massive consumption of meat. **Intensive farming is not only expensive in terms of water resources, but it is also the main cause of greenhouse gas emissions** released during the digestion and decomposition of bovine manure, as well as deforestation and soil erosion due to the search for new lands to cultivate animal feed such as soy. In particular, a report by the FAO (Food and Agriculture Organization of the United Nations, 2021) highlights that **livestock production** accounts for 14.2% of total greenhouse gas emissions from human activities, of which 65% is caused solely by beef and dairy cattle farming.

To reduce these issues, it would be enough to change eating habits worldwide towards **healthy and sustainable dietary regimes based on whole grains, legumes, fruits, vegetables, nuts, and seeds.** If demand for high environmental impact foods such as meat and other animal products were immediately contained in favor of equally nutrient-rich and healthier plant-based solutions, it would indeed be possible not only to **drastically reduce emissions but also to increase food production significantly using the same resources.** In fact, the production of animal products such as red meat (especially beef and pork) and dairy products (especially cattle) requires much more land and water than plant-based alternatives, even for the same energy and nutritional content, not only for the maintenance of the animals themselves but also for the production of feed during breeding.

It is estimated that if the global population made more responsible food choices, thanks to the implementation of **advanced techniques such as precision agriculture and minimal use of water,** the global production system would be able **to meet the caloric needs of the entire population,** even in the case of a prospective increase in the world's population. This aspect is particularly relevant in relation to the inequality of the **redistribution of food resources** among the population of high-income countries, where according to WHO data from 2016, 2.5

out of 10 people are overweight (about 2 billion worldwide, of which 650,000 are obese), and that of poor countries, where 1 out of 10 people suffer from malnutrition (more than 820 million worldwide).

Lifestyle and Environment

After the fossil fuel and food production industries, **motorized transportation is among the most polluting factors in the world.** Therefore, to reduce greenhouse gases, it is necessary to drastically modify our travel habits. This is suggested by a study promoted by the EU and published in the journal "Global Environmental Change" (2021). Supported by the PASTA project and funded by the EU, the study analyzed seven European cities: Antwerp (Belgium), Barcelona (Spain), London (UK), Orebro (Sweden), Rome (Italy), Vienna (Austria) and Zurich (Switzerland). The research shows that personal carbon emissions in cities can be significantly **reduced up to a quarter simply by replacing a car trip with a walk, bike ride, or electric bike ride.** In conclusion, eating and living in a healthy and sustainable way, and walking are some habits that we could adopt to contribute to the environment and its health, as well as for our own benefit.

7.9.   STRATEGY 7: FOLLOW THE EXAMPLE OF BLUE ZONE CENTENARIANS

There are some areas in the world characterized by a very long-lived population. The most famous are the "Blue Zones," a term used to identify a geographic area where life expectancy is higher than the world average, described by *New York Times* journalist Dan Buettner in a 2005 article for *National Geographic.* These include **Okinawa in Japan, the Nicoya Peninsula in Costa Rica, the island of Ikaria in Greece, the eastern coast of Sardinia in the Ogliastra area of Italy, and the Seventh-day Adventist community in Loma Linda, California.**

Buettner and many other scientists who have dedicated themselves to studying centenarians in these areas, such as Valter

Longo, indicate that in these places one can live longer and healthier thanks to a lifestyle based on some important rules to follow, starting with **a semi-vegetarian diet** with consumption of legumes with many complex carbohydrates, a lot of nuts, a little fish, few proteins, few sugars, and few saturated and trans fats. Many of these centenarians **eat at most 2-3 times a day, with a small meal in the evening, often before it gets dark.** They generally tend to consume a limited variety of foods, typical of their land, although in some cases they follow more varied diets. For example, the inhabitants of Okinawa once consumed most of their calories from purple sweet potatoes, which is now much less common.

In addition to these elements, there is **moderate consumption of calories and alcoholic beverages, constant and measured physical activity,** little or no **smoking, little stress,** the idea of **family as the center of one's existence,** feeling **socially useful,** having a full and **fulfilling social and spiritual life,** and above all, feeling that one has a **purpose in life.** In fact, in addition to important variables such as genetic factors, nutrition, physical exercise, and lifestyle, Professor Longo, after listening to numerous stories told by centenarians from all over the world, many of which were very different, noticed a common denominator: the sense of purpose in life, **the will to live.**

"My colleague Jim Vaupel, Director of the Max-Planck Institute for Demography, once proposed a revelation that surprised me. 'What I have discovered was that many of the world's oldest people have in common is their **tenacity.** They are fighters, capable of surviving even the death of their own children, as happened to Madame Calment, the French woman who set the record of 122 years, or the Italian Emma Morano, who reached the age of 117.' It is said that Madame Calment always said, 'If you can't do anything about it, don't worry about it,' and that, to a journalist who hoped to see her again the following year, she replied with spirit, 'Why? You don't look sick!'"

It is difficult to quantify tenacity and the will to live in scientific terms. What we can say is that some centenarians find their strength in God, others in their families, and many in the simple joy of living, made up of small moments such as enjoying a sweet, after going through world wars and famines, when this was not possible. (Adapted from Valter Longo, *The Longevity Diet,* p. 95-6, 99).

8. RECIPES

8.1. RECIPES TO COMPOSE

COLD PORRIDGE

Ingredients for 1 person
Preparation time: 15 min + rest overnight in the fridge
Difficulty: easy

Ingredients

- ½ cup whole oat flakes
- ½ cup of almond milk or another plant-based milk as preferred
- "Fatty" toppings such as nuts, seeds, nut butter, or dark chocolate
- Toppings with "sugars" such as jam, fresh fruit, honey, or agave syrup

Preparation

In a small bowl, combine the oats, plant-based milk, and other spices to taste, such as cinnamon and some seeds or dried fruit.

Mix and add a spoonful of jam inside.

Melt the dark chocolate and cover the porridge (if you want to use chocolate).

Place in the refrigerator overnight.

In the morning, the chocolate (if you have chosen this as your fat) will have solidified and will make a tasty coat.

This is a tasty recipe for a healthy and nutritious summer breakfast.

SMOOTHIE

Ingredients for 1 person
Preparation time: 3 min
Difficulty: easy

Ingredients

- 1 cup frozen strawberries, blueberries, and/or bananas
- 1 cup of coconut milk or another plant-based milk
- 1 tablespoon honey
- 1 tablespoon ground flax seeds (or others)
- coconut flakes as a garnish

Preparation

Blend all the ingredients.

If you prefer less thick smoothies, add more coconut milk or any other liquid.

If you prefer them thicker, you can use peanut butter (without sugar) or plant-based yogurt.

To taste, you can always add spices such as cinnamon, turmeric, ginger, bitter cocoa powder, coffee, etc.

FETTAMISÙ WITH PLANT-BASED YOGURT, RASPBERRIES AND DARK CHOCOLATE

Ingredients for 1 person
Preparation time: 5 min
Difficulty: easy

Ingredients

- 3 rusks (dry biscuit)
- 1 cup of coconut milk or another plant-based milk
- 1 cup raspberries
- 125 g (5 oz) of plant-based yogurt
- 30 g (1 oz) of dark chocolate >85%

Preparation

The night before, dip the 3 rusks in the plant-based milk.

Make layers interspersed with yogurt and raspberries.

Melt the dark chocolate.

Use it to cover this tower of rusks.

8.2. SNACK RECIPES

APRICOT STUFFED WITH HAZELNUT CREAM AND A GLASS OF PLANT-BASED MILK

Ingredients for 1 person
Preparation time: 5 min
Difficulty: easy

Ingredients

- 150 g (5 oz) of apricots or other fruit depending on the season, for example pears, bananas, and raspberries
- 100% hazelnut cream, i.e., a spreadable cream whose only ingredient is hazelnuts.

Preparation

Wash the fruit.

Cut it in half.

Remove the stone (if present).

The space left by the stone (or the surface of the fruit cut in half) will be filled with a spoonful of 100% hazelnut cream.

The cream alone can be slightly bitter, especially in comparison to other industrial creams rich in sugars.

However, the combination with fruit, which is naturally sweet, will allow for a truly pleasant flavor.

For a complete snack, also combine with plant-based milk, such as coconut.

DELICIOUS SNACK BARS

** The help of an adult is required*

Ingredients for six bars
Preparation time: 40 minutes plus cooling time
Difficulty: easy

Ingredients

- 50 g (1.7 oz) of hazelnuts
- 100 g (3.5) of muesli
- 2 tablespoons of honey
- 50 g (1.7 oz) of dark chocolate

Preparation

Toast and chop 50 g / 1.7 oz of hazelnuts for two minutes in a pan. You must absolutely avoid burning them, which is harmful to your health.

Mix them with 100 g / 3.5 oz of muesli and 2 tablespoons of honey.

Mix and place the mixture on a baking tray, covered with baking paper. Better in a rectangular mold, to have a precise shape. Level and compact with your hands or a spoon.

Bake in a preheated oven at 170° C / 338 ° F for 15-20 minutes.

Once the mixture is warm, cut into equal rectangles with the classic snack bar shape. Use a large knife oiled with olive oil. Allow the snack bars to cool completely, perhaps placing them in the fridge for 20-30 minutes.

Melt 50 g / 1.7 oz of dark chocolate in a bain-marie. Dip the snack bar 1/4 of the way into the chocolate to create the base.

Put them back in the fridge to cool completely. You can keep them for 3-4 days wrapped in a little baking paper.

PERSIMMON (OR BANANA, OR AVOCADO) PUDDING AND CHOCOLATE

Ingredients for one person
Preparation time: 5 min
Difficulty: easy

Ingredients

- 100 g (3.5 oz) of persimmons or banana or avocado
  1 medium-sized fruit)
- 50-100 ml (3.5 -6 tbsp) of plant-based milk
- Bitter cocoa powder
- 1 tablespoon honey (if you are using avocado)

Preparation

Using a blender, mix the persimmon, banana, or avocado pieces well.

Add approximately 50-100 ml (3.5 -6 tbsp) of plant-based milk if the mixture is too dry and not blended.

Add the bitter cocoa powder (2 tablespoons for each fruit)

If using avocado, add a spoonful of honey to sweeten.

In the case of persimmons and bananas, there is no need to sweeten because these two fruits are naturally sweet.

It should be stored in the refrigerator for a maximum of 3 days.

TOAST WITH FIGS AND RICOTTA

Ingredients for one person
Preparation time: 5 min
Difficulty: easy

Ingredients

- 1-2 slices of toasted bread
- 20 g (0.7 oz) of fresh ricotta
- 2-3 figs or other fruits

Preparation

All you need to do is toast some bread, preferably whole wheat and perhaps also rich in seeds.

Sprinkle on fresh ricotta and some figs cut in half or other fruits, depending on the season (e.g., grapes, pears, peaches, etc.)

RICE CAKE WITH CHICKPEA HUMMUS AND TOMATOES

Ingredients for one person
Preparation time: 5 min
Difficulty: easy

Ingredients

- 240 g (8.5 oz) of chickpeas
- Juice of half a lemon
- 2 tablespoons of tahini or EVO oil (Extra Virgin Olive Oil)
- 1 pinch of cumin (to taste)
- 3 whole wheat rice cakes
- 4-5 cherry tomatoes
- Oregano to taste

Preparation

Chickpea hummus can be prepared on the spot, or beforehand. Simply blend some pre-cooked chickpeas with a little of the preserving/cooking water (e.g., 240 g or 1 cup), the juice of half a lemon, 2 tablespoons of tahini or EVO oil, and a pinch of cumin, if desired.

This very simple hummus is excellent spread on whole wheat rice cakes and sprinkled with cherry tomatoes cut in half and seasoned with oregano.

9. CONCLUSION

We have reached the end of this manual which has guided us through the principles of a healthy lifestyle, balanced nutrition, and the importance of physical exercise.

Share this knowledge with children, so that they can grow up aware and make choices that will lead them to a long and healthy life.

Each one of you can help build a community that promotes health and well-being for all. Continue to be positive examples and to be bearers of change.

Together we can make a difference in the lives and present and future health of many! Thank you for being part of this journey.

10. ACKNOWLEDGMENTS

We would like to express our deepest gratitude to the people who made possible the creation of "Nutrition Begins as Children" and the manual for families and teachers.

First, we want to extend a warm thank you to the artist Manuela Lupis, whose creative skills and extraordinary illustrations made the book visually fascinating and engaging.

Heartfelt thanks go to Cristina Villa, Program Director at the Valter Longo Foundation and collaborator of the Create Cures Foundation, who played a fundamental role in supervising the project and writing the manual.

Thanks to Romina Inès Cervigni, Chief Scientific Officer of the Valter Longo Foundation and collaborator of the Create Cures Foundation, for providing a solid knowledge base and for ensuring that the contents were accurate and informative.

Thanks to everyone who made this book possible. We are grateful for your support.

Finally, we thank you, our readers, for giving us the opportunity to share this information with you. We hope that this book has been useful to you and that you have gained inspiration and knowledge from it.

Valter Longo Foundation

11. BIBLIOGRAPHY

ADI - X Giornata del Fiocchetto Lilla: Disturbi alimentari: nell'anno della pandemia aumentano i casi tra i giovanissimi. 15 marzo 2021. Da: https://www.adiitalia.org/video-trailer/video-trailer-5/2021.html

Almirante P. "Obesità e depressione per un bambino su due: il lascito del Covid". La tecnica della scuola. 03-06-2021. Da: https://www.tecnicadellascuola.it/obesita-e-depressione-per-un-bambino-su-due-il-lascito-del-covid

Amati C. "Valter Longo: «La dieta mediterranea è stata snaturata, fatta così fa male»." Cook Corriere. 16-11-2020. Da: https://www.corriere.it/cook/news/20_novembre_16/valter-longo-la-dieta-mediterranea-stata-snaturata-fatta-cosi-fa-male-2c99fe1c-2684-11eb-bd3c-8e368a362c56.shtml

Associazione Italiana di Oncologia Medica. "Tumori: Un milione e 400mila screening in meno nei primi 5 mesi del 2020. Rischio di diagnosi più avanzate, servono risorse per la telemedicina." 24-09-2020. Da: https://www.aiom.it/speciale-covid-19-tumori-un-milione-400mila-screening-in-meno-primi-5-mesi-2020-rischio-diagnosi-avanzate-servono-risorse-per-telemedicina/

Belvedere V., Grando A. *Sustainable Operations and Supply Chain Management*. Wiley. 2017.

Italian Obesity Barometer Report 2022 – dati IBDO Foundation in collaborazione con ISTAT, Coreresearch e BHAVE. https://issuu.com/raffaelecreativagroupcom/docs/italian_obesity_barometer_report_2022

Brand C. et Al. "The climate change mitigation impacts of active travel: Evidence from a longitudinal panel study in seven European cities". *Global Environmental Change*, Volume 67, 2021.

Consiglio per la ricerca in agricoltura e l'analisi dell'economia agraria. "Covid-19: come sono cambiate le nostre abitudini alimentari durante il lockdown?" 26-05-2020. Da: https://www.crea.gov.it/-/covid-19-come-sono-cambiate-le-nostre-abitudini-alimentari-durante-il-lockdown-

D'Aria I. "L'Oms: l'80% degli adolescenti non fa abbastanza attività fisica." 21-11-2019. La Repubblica. Da: https://www.repubblica.it/salute/alimentazione-e-fitness/2019/11/21/news/oms_1_80_degli_adolescenti_non_fa_abbastanza_attivita_fisica-241525259/

EpiCentro Istituto Superiore di Sanità. "Caratteristiche dei pazienti deceduti positivi all'infezione da SARS-CoV-2 in Italia." Da: https://www.epicentro.iss.it/coronavirus/sars-cov-2-decessi-italia

European Everyday of Sport. "Don't skip gym: Physical education important to learning, academic success." 2017. Da: https://m.eusport.org/news/beactive_news_section/dont_skip_gym_physical_education_important_learning

FAO - Key Facts and Findings. By the numbers: GHG emissions by livestock. Consultato il 10-8-21. Da: http://www.fao.org/news/story/en/item/197623/icode/

Fornili M, Petri D, Berrocal C, Fiorentino G, Ricceri F, Macciotta A, Bruno A, Farinella D, Baccini M, Severi G, Baglietto L. "Psychological distress in the academic population and its association with socio-demographic and lifestyle characteristics during COVID-19 pandemic lockdown: Results from a large multicenter Italian study". PLOS ONE. 10-03-2021. Da: https://journals.plos.org/plosone/article?id=10.1371/journal.pone.0248370

Gascon M., Götschi T., de Nazelle A., Gracia E., Ambròs A., Márquez S., Marquet O., Avila-Palencia I., Brand C., Iacorossi F., Raser E., Gaupp-Berghausen M., Dons E., Laeremans M., Kahlmeier S., Sánchez J., Gerike R., Anaya-Boig E., Int Panis L. e Nieuwenhuijsen M. "Correlates of Walking for Travel in Seven European Cities: The PASTA Project." Environmental Health Perspective, 127(9). 18-09-2019. Da: https://ehp.niehs.nih.gov/doi/10.1289/EHP4603

Howell B. "Top 7 Most Polluting Industries." The Eco Experts. 29-04-2021. Da: https://www.theecoexperts.co.uk/blog/top-7-most-polluting-industries

IBDO Foundation. "Obesity Monitor: Monitoring prevention, cure, political, social and economic facts on obesity care." *1st Italian Obesity Barometer Report*. 2019. Da: http://www.ibdo.it/pdf/OBESITY-REPORT-2019.pdf

International Diabetes Federation. "Diabetes Atlas Seventh Edition." 2015. Da: https://www.diabetesatlas.org/upload/resources/previous/files/7/IDF%20Diabetes%20Atlas%207th.pdf

IPSOS: Diet & Health Under Covid-19. January 2021. Da: https://www.ipsos.com/sites/default/files/ct/news/documents/2021-01/diet-and-health-under-covid-19_0.pdf

Istat. "Prima Ondata della Pandemia. Un'analisi della mortalità per cause e luogo del decesso. Marzo-Aprile 2020." 21-04-2021. Da: https://www.istat.it/it/files/2021/04/Report-Cause-di-Morte_21_04_2021.pdf

Longo V. *La dieta della longevità*. Milano• Vallardi. 2016./ *Alla tavola della longevità* (2017)/ *La longevità inizia da bambini* (2019)

Meridiano Sanità. "Rapporto 2018." Da: https://www.sanita24.ilsole24ore.com/pdf2010/Editrice/ILSOLE24ORE/QUOTIDIANO_SANITA/Online/_Oggetti_Correlati/Documenti/2018/11/14/MeridianoSanita2018.pdf?uuid=AE922sfG

Ministero della Salute. "La Situazione Sanitaria del Paese", Quadro Generale, Impatto delle Malattie (1.5). https://www.salute.gov.it/rssp/paginaParagrafoRssp.jsp?sezione=situazione&capitolo=quadro&id=2646

Nardone P., Pierannunzio D., Ciardullo S., Spinelli A., Donati S., Cavallo F., Dalmasso P., Vieno A., Lazzeri G., Galeone D. "La Sorveglianza HBSC 2018 - Health Behaviour in School-aged Children: risultati dello studio italiano tra i ragazzi di 11, 13 e 15 anni." Istituto Superiore di Sanità. 2020. Da: https://www.iss.it/

documents/20126/0/HBSC.pdf/97b1cfee-444c-bfd4-ab58-d0b-1dcb504fb?t=1603882812589

OERSA/ REA. "Cambiamenti delle abitudini alimentari nell'EMERGENZA COVID-19". https://www.crea.gov.it/-/covid-19-come-sono-cambiate-le-nostre-abitudini-alimentari-durante-il-lockdown-

Save the Children. "L'impatto del coronavirus sulla povertà educativa". Da: https://s3.savethechildren.it/public/files/uploads/pubblicazioni/limpatto-del-coronavirus-sulla-poverta-educativa_0.pdf

Società Italiana di Nutrizione Umana (SINU) - IV Revisione dei Livelli di Assunzione di Riferimento di Nutrienti ed energia per la popolazione italiana (LARN), 2014. Da: https://sinu.it/tabelle-larn-2014/

Spinelli A. et Al. Prevalence of Severe Obesity among Primary School Children in 21 European Countries. *Karger*. Maggio 2019. Da: https://www.karger.com/Article/FullText/500436#

The EAT-Lancet Commission on Food, Planet, Health. "Can we feed a future population of 10 billion people a healthy diet within planetary boundaries?" Da: https://eatforum.org/eat-lancet-commission/

The Intergovernmental Panel on Climate Change. "Climate change and land." *Special report*. Da: https://www.ipcc.ch/srccl/

Unicef. "The State of Food Security and Nutrition in the World 2019." 07-2019. Da: https://data.unicef.org/resources/sofi-2019/

United Nations Department of Economic and Social Affairs. "The 17 goals". Da: https://sdgs.un.org/goals

WCFC and AICR, "Diet, Nutrition, Physical Activity, and Cancer: a Global Perspective". Da: https://www.wcrf.org/wp-content/uploads/2021/02/Summary-of-Third-Expert-Report-2018.pdf

World Health Organization, "Healty Diet", aggiornato 2021. Da: https://www.who.int/news-room/fact-sheets/detail/healthy-diet

World Health Organization Factsheet, "Malnutrition". 9 June 2021. Da: https://www.who.int/news-room/fact-sheets/detail/malnutrition

World Health Organization Factsheet, "Obesity and Overweight". 9 June 2021. Da: https://www.who.int/news-room/fact-sheets/detail/obesity-and-overweight

World Health Organization Regional Office for Europe. "Data and statistics: The challenge of obesity - quick statistics." Da: https://www.euro.who.int/en/health-topics/noncommunicable-diseases/obesity/data-and-statistics

World Health Organization. "Physical Activity." 2022. https://www.who.int/news-room/fact-sheets/detail/physical-activity

www.ingramcontent.com/pod-product-compliance
Lightning Source LLC
Chambersburg PA
CBHW050850260726
48660CB00006B/2557